Paleo Diet for Beginners:

The 21-Day Challenge to Eating Healthy and Losing Weight

Emma S. Fisher

Legal & Disclaimer

The information contained in this book has been provided for educational and entertainment purposes only and is not designed to replace any form of medicine or professional medical advice.

The information contained in this book has been compiled from sources deemed reliable, and it is accurate to the best of the Author's knowledge. The Author asks all customers to consult their doctor for professional medical advice, any concerns, and personal requirements with this diet. Every person and body is different, so be sure your doctor approves before you attempt this diet. Emma Fisher and associates are not liable to any complications with this diet guide.

Table of Contents

Introduction

Conclusion

Introduction

I am quite certain that even before you've decided to try the Paleo diet and downloaded this book, you've heard and read something about this popular diet. It's probably because a lot of Hollywood celebrities, athletes, and other popular personalities have endorsed this diet and swear that Paleo has helped them achieve their health goals. Also, since the diet was introduced to the market, its followers and the people who are curious about the diet is continuously growing; in fact, in 2013, the Paleo Diet was named as the top searched diet plan by Google that year.

But what is the Paleo Diet anyway? How can "eating like the cavemen did" help achieve your health goals? What are the foods that are Paleo-friendly? These are the questions that this book will answer.

Before I go on, let me thank you for downloading this book "Paleo Diet for Beginners:The 21-Day Challenge to Eating Healthy and Losing Weight". Through the chapters of this book, you will learn why Paleo is one of the top diets of this generation. You will understand how the "modern man's diet" has caused man to regress from being agile, athletic, and lean into being sluggish, inactive, and overweight and why going Paleo is the solution to achieving your goals such as eating healthy and losing weight.

I've entitled this book as the "21-Day challenge" because 21 days is just enough for you to begin turning your back to your eating habits and ultimately live a Paleo lifestyle. Do not worry, Paleo is not a crash diet where you have to starve yourself in order to reap its benefits; in fact going Paleo Diet means you're going to eat three meals a day, even with snacks in between! And the best thing is that you're still going to achieve your health goals if you stick with the foods that are Paleo-approved (which I will discuss in one chapter of this book).

In addition, to guide you in this journey, a chapter in this book is dedicated to help you effectively transit from your old diet to Paleo. Trust me, just give it 21 days and you'll surely be on your way to a healthier life!

Lastly, three chapters of this book are delicious Paleo recipes (from breakfast, snacks, and main meals) that you could use on the first week of your Paleo journey.

Are you all set for the challenge? Begin right away to see the results everyone is enjoying!

Chapter 1

Paleo Diet 101

Most people today live a fast-paced life. Day in and day out we juggle different responsibilities, between our families, our work and our social life and in the end, we often forget that we must also take care of our body. We become unmindful of what we eat, often opting for food that are "instant" or "fast" and also neglect to allot time for exercise or other physical activities.

Although we think that this lifestyle makes us more productive, what most people tend to forget is that careless eating and being inactive could lead to bigger bellies, drained energy, and a whole lot of health problems.

While exercising could help you gain more energy and shed weight, the most important thing that you have to focus on if you want to live a healthy lifestyle is your diet. That's because the nutrients and vitamins that you consume from your food are those that your body utilizes in order for it to become in top shape! Do you want to lose weight? Assess your diet! Remember, weight loss is 70% diet and 30% exercise.

What's wrong with my diet?

If you try to imagine and compare what cavemen looked like and how an average man looks today, how will you describe them? I'm sure you're thinking that cavemen are those who have lean bodies, are agile and fast runners (because they hunt their food), while modern man is someone who has

1

flabs, is sluggish, and easily tired. But what could be the reason why man turned from someone who has abs to someone who has a big belly? That's right! DIET!

Proponents of the Paleo Diet believe that "modern diet", characterized to be rich in carbohydrates, sugar, unhealthy fat, and additives is the reason why man's physique has regressed over the years.

The Agricultural Era, in particular, is what the followers of Paleo identified as the main contributor to why a lot of people are at risk of "diseases of civilization" such as obesity, hypertension, diabetes, and different types of cancers. From consuming foods that are rich in protein (cavemen ate a lot of meat), healthy fats, and fiber (from fruits and vegetables), man became dependent on farm-raised foods such as grains, bread, and pasta which are all carb-rich foods. As you know a high-carb diet could contribute to weight gain because any carbohydrate that is not burned as energy (in the form of glucose) turns into body fat. Also, our cavemen ancestors were more athletic and energetic than modern man, because they had to gather and hunt for their food. In contrary, when farming and agriculture were discovered, men moved forward from growing crops and raising animals as an easier food source.

Although our means of eating food have evolved throughout the centuries, the followers of Paleo believe that the problem is that our genetic make-up haven't actually adapted to modern man's diet. This means that our bodies are still not accustomed to farmed and carb-rich foods which are mostly available today. The agricultural era made us believe that in order to satiate our hunger, we need to munch on grains, rice, and other foods rich in carbohydrates; which is a far cry to man's original diet which is high in protein, healthy fat, and fiber.

Junk Food and the Body

To make matters worse, it's not only the high-carb foods that we all should worry about. "Instant foods"—those that come in cans, ready to eat boxes, fast foods, etc. are also contributors to man's poor health.

These junk or empty calorie foods have high contents of sugar, sodium, and fat that can lead to obesity and many health problems including arthritis, diabetes, hypertension that could cause serious heart problems. These foods do not contain any nutrient value that our body needs to keep us healthy. It could only make us feel chronically exhausted which will not, in any way, help us accomplish our daily tasks. The high content of sugar in junk food also puts our metabolism under stress; consuming refined sugar triggers our pancreas to produce high amounts of insulin which is dangerous to our body.

Junk food also contains a great amount of fat (the bad kind of fat). And when this accumulates in our body, we will add on weight that can lead to obesity. The more weight we gain, the more we become at risk for severe and chronic illnesses like arthritis, type 2 diabetes, hypertension, arterial plaque build-up that leads to high cholesterol, and heart diseases that may even lead to the deadly heart attack.

3

The high amount of fat can also lead to poor concentration because of the lack of oxygen we are getting. It can not only damage our heart, but also the liver. The high content of trans-fatty acids in junk foods can lead to fatty deposits that can result to liver dysfunction.

Too much sodium in our body can also lead to renal malfunction, leading to kidney disease. Studies also show that high sodium-diet is one of the main contributors to hypertension—a condition that could lead to other more serious health problems.

The Paleo Solution

Like as said in the introduction, whether your goal is to lose weight, prevent health problems, or to ultimately live and eat healthy, the Paleo Diet is the answer to help you achieve those goals.

Also known as the "Caveman's Diet" or the "Stone Age Diet", Paleo's principle is simple: avoid any type of foods that were not available during the Paleolithic Era. This is because Paleo proponents believe that modern man's diet (which is made of grains, sweets, processed food, etc.) is the factor that is causing harm to the body.

What's the solution? Eat all-natural food, such as grass-fed meat, wild-caught fish, organically grown produce, etc. Anything that contains grains, preservatives, sugar, and salt should be avoided.

Although Paleo was only put into the spotlight in the year

2000's through Dr. Loren Cordain, founder of the Paleo movement, a lot of research in the past could attest to the health claims of the Paleo diet.

In 1913, a man named Joseph Knowles was able to come up with a healthier diet after living like a hunter-gatherer in the wilderness for two months. Knowles claims that he felt stronger and healthier after living like that of our cavemen ancestors.

Decades after gastroenterologist Dr. Walter L. Voegtlin published a book "The Stone Age Diet" where he first coined the term "Paleo Diet" he suggests that 99.9% of modern man's genetic code came from cavemen, which means that our bodies will naturally strive on a diet that our hunter-gatherer ancestors ate. This breakthrough was followed by a lot more scientific studies about the diet.

These studies only prove that following a diet patterned over the caveman's diet, you are not only able to lose weight and achieve a body like the cavemen, but you can also prevent numerous diseases brought about poor food choices.

Paleo Health Benefits

Paleo diet as we now all know advocates to consume all-natural food such as grass-fed animals, free range fowls (chicken, turkey, duck and the likes), wild-caught fish (not the ones grown from the fish pens), organic eggs, nuts, tubers, fruits and vegetables. Therefore, a Paleo meal is far more nutritious than any fast food and processed food you can buy from the grocery.

- Meat from grass-fed animal is high in Omega 3 fatty acids that are good for the heart.

- Free range-fowls have less fat and are free from antibiotics which is unsafe to eat.

- Wild-caught fish is free from mercury and toxins compared to farmed fish.

- Fruits and vegetables are high in fiber content which is needed by our body to produce good microorganisms that aids our stomach to digest our food well.

Aside from eating a healthy diet, here are the other benefits one can get from this diet:

1. Lose weight—Paleo diet is proven to help shed off excess fat in the body. This high-protein diet is sure to help you achieve a "bikini perfect bod"

2. Lesser risk of developing serious health diseases—as you cut down your junk food consumption and other unhealthy food that causes harm you also reduce the risk of having dreadful diseases. The healthier the food you eat, the more nutrients you get; the more it makes you fit, agile, and healthy.

3. Improved absorption and digestion of food—since you now consume more of fruits and vegetables that are high in fiber, the digestive system can now function well. This means that the nutrients and vitamins in our food can now be properly absorbed and utilize by our body.

4. Eating "clean" food— since Paleo advocates all-natural

food, the diet enables you to eat with no preservatives and other chemicals that are toxic to the body.

5. Eat food rich in Iron— Iron is very important in our body because it carries oxygen to the blood stream. People with iron deficiency tend to have anemia, which can lead to a type of cancer called leukemia if not properly addressed.

6. Keeps you satiated—Proper combination of healthy fat and fiber from meat and, fruits and vegetables will keep you feeling full for a longer period of time. That means you are able to curb your cravings and unnecessary trips to the pantry, which could ultimately help you lose weight.

7. Counting calories is not required—Paleo diet is easy and simple to follow. Since you will just focus on natural and healthy foods, you can eat anything until you're full as long as it's a combination of red meat, fruits and vegetables. There's no need to painstakingly monitor your calories in this diet.

Paleo diet is easy as 1-2-3 and you can choose from an array of Paleo approved foods. Turn to the next chapter to learn how to shop the Paleo way!

Chapter 2

The Paleo Shopping Cart

What is great about the Paleo Diet is that even though you follow a healthier diet, it doesn't mean that it limits you to only a number of food types. In fact, you will realize that Paleo offers a variety of foods that you can enjoy. Here is a comprehensive list of Paleo-friendly foods.

- **Protein foods**- when purchasing this type of meat, keep in mind to buy only the naturally grown (organic) or grass-fed meats. You can also buy frozen meat, but the rule of the thumb is avoiding processed food.

<u>Meat and Poultry Products</u>

- o Pork chops
- o Tenderloin
- o Sirloin steak
- o Beef steak
- o Lean ground beef
- o Lean ground pork
- o Bacon (Yes! That's right!)
- o Chicken meat (organic or free-range)
- o Turkey or duck Quail
- o Lamb
- o Rabbit
- o Organic Eggs (you'll eat a lot in this diet!)

Fish

- o Tuna
- o Bass
- o Salmon
- o Mackerel
- o Eel

- o Red Snapper
- o Trout
- o Cod
- o Tilapia

Shell Fish

- o Oyster
- o Lobster
- o Mussels
- o Crab
- o Shrimp
- o Clams

- o Scallops
- o Crayfish
- o Prawn

- **Carbohydrates** —Paleo Diet is a low-carbohydrate diet, but it doesn't mean that you have to completely cut it off in your diet. You can get carbs not by eating grains, but from consuming a whole lot of fruits and vegetables.

Fruits

- o Mango
- o Cherries
- o Papaya
- o Strawberries
- o Blueberries

- o Blackberries
- o Honeydew
- o Watermelon
- o Cantaloupe
- o Kiwi

- Lime or lemon
- Avocado
- Coconut
- Peaches

Vegetables

- Pumpkin
- Cucumber
- Squash
- Turnips
- Beets
- Zucchini
- Carrots
- Tomatoes
- Celery
- Green bell Pepper
- Red bell pepper
- Radish
- Cabbage
- Lettuce
- Kale
- Cauliflower
- Artichoke
- Asparagus
- Spinach

- **Herbs and Spices** – below are the list of herbs and spices you can use to spice up your dishes
  - Black Pepper
  - Cumin
  - Basil
  - Chili powder
  - Cilantro
  - Curry

- **Fats** –not all fats are bad for the health. There are also good sources of fat.

Nuts and Seeds

- Brazilian Nuts
- Sesame Seeds
- Almonds
- Walnuts
- Sunflower Seeds
- Macadamia
- Hazel
- Pumpkin
- Sunflower Seeds

Oils

- Walnut oil
- Coconut oil
- Olive oil
- Avocado oil
- Canola oil

Below are the food types you must avoid in a Paleo Diet

- **Grains and Legumes**
  - Cereals
  - Peanuts
  - Rice

- **Processed foods** – avoid instant foods
  - Sausages
  - Canned goods
  - Nuggets
  - Hotdogs
  - Microwaveable foods
  - Instant noodles

- **Dairy Foods**

  o Yoghurt
  o Ice cream
  o Butter
  o Cheese
  o Milk (low-fat, skimmed, whole, powdered)

- **Beverages**

  o All types of sodas
  o Energy drinks
  o Coffee
  o Artificially flavored juices

- Fast food

- Salt and other Salty Food

- Sugar

- Refined Vegetable Oils

Chapter 3

Transitioning to Paleo

Before starting any diet it's important that you are convicted that you like what you're doing, and you're doing it for yourself and your loved ones. Saying "Yes I will start doing it!" is the first step to a lifestyle change. This will help you get through the 21-day challenge before eating and living Paleo will become natural to you.

But before you begin, I'd like to give you a few tips in order for you to successfully follow the Paleo Lifestyle.

Tips to Successful Follow the Paleo Lifestyle

1. **Commit to the Diet**—deciding to commit yourself to this diet, or should I say lifestyle, is not an easy task. But with the proper determination, you will be able to take control of your life. You can easily break your eating habits and focus on your goal to be fit and lose weight if you commit yourself to the diet.

Many people have tried this and became successful; if they were able to do it, you can do it too!

2. **Clean Out Your Food Cupboard**—emptying your cupboard is an evident act that you are serious in following the Paleo Lifestyle. Assess your pantry, refrigerator and any other food storage boxes and

remove any junk food, sweets, pastries, bread and any other food that is not in the list of Paleo diet (refer to chapter 2 for the list).

Cleaning out your food storage will also keep you away from being tempted to go back to your old habit of eating these junk foods again. You can either dump them into the garbage bin, or donate them to the needy. They would sure benefit from it.

3. **Devote for Time and Resources**— since Paleo Diet is a lifestyle change, it is a must that you devote your time in learning new things about this diet. You must also be willing to spend more time in the kitchen as well as buy equipment that you may need in preparing your meals. Looking for food market and supermarkets that sells best Paleo food is also a must.

4. **Plan the Timing**—scheduling the time when to start the Paleo Diet is very important. Do not start during Christmas holidays, and big events like family reunions because you may be tempted to eat food that is not on your Paleo list.

People around you may influence you, since you have not yet established your habit of eating Paleo foods.

5. **Look for a Support Group**—having someone to guide and help you during the period of dieting and establishing your lifestyle is very crucial. Tell someone closest to you like your spouse, best friend, your housemates or a support group that is into the Paleo diet. You could also ask them to face the 21-day Paleo

Challenge with you!

At the start, you may feel frustrated and discouraged but having someone to motivate and encourage you and somebody you can voice out your frustrations, fears and stress can help you lessen your load.

6. Record Your Milestones—consult your doctor or a health care provider especially when you are under medication before starting this diet. It is but proper that a professional doctor or a health provider can guide you properly.

After doing this, keep a record in your notebook the initial measurements of your weight, waistline and even your BMI (Body Mass Index). Then start recording your milestones as you go on with your diet. At the end of your dieting period you can make comparisons on how you have progressed. This record can also serve as a motivation to keep you going when you see how far you've achieved in your health goals.

7. **Make Your List Readily Available**—a list that is always available will make your shopping much easier and will help you chose the healthy food the Paleo way. Stick to this list and avoid any aisles in the grocery that isn't included in the list.

8. **Set Your Specific Goal**—set a realistic goal before starting the Paleo Diet to see the success of your weight loss. One pound of weight loss a week can be a good start.

9. **Avoid Eating Out**--Refrain from going to restaurants to avoid temptation. Instead, prepare your meals at home and share it with your love ones, that way they too may be

encourage to start dieting too. You can start creating your meal plans with the recipes, this I will share with you in the next chapters.

10. **Do Not Give Up**— if you fail, start all over again. This can happen when you are just starting. There will be times that you will be tempted to try some "unhealthy foods". If this is the case, don't lose hope, get back and carry on. Just remember this cliché "If others can to it, I can do it myself."

Now that I've given you some tips to help you start, now is the time to begin your 21-day Paleo Challenge! Turn to the next chapter and see what challenges awaits!

Chapter 4

The 21-Day Paleo Challenge

In the previous chapters, you learned about the basics of the Paleo Diet, what type of foods you should have in your pantry and some tips on how you can transit into the diet. In this chapter, I want you to buckle up as you go through the challenges I listed down in this chapter. Of course, you can create your own version of a 21-day challenge and use this chapter as guide.

The Magic Number 21

I'm pretty sure you've heard that it takes 21 days to make or break a habit, but where did this idea come from?

In the 1960's Dr. Maxwell Maltz, an American cosmetic surgeon, published a book entitled Psycho-Cybernetics. This book discussed Dr. Maltz' observation about how his patients were able to adjust to changes in a period of 21 days or more. According to this book, his patients who underwent operations such as rhinoplasty (nose job) or breast augmentation were able to adjust to the changes in their body after 21 days. He also observed his behavior and how he was able to adapt to changes after 21 days. His idea was so revolutionary that a number of self-help books were written based on his suggestion.

However, I would like you to remember that you cannot (magically) change a habit *in* 21 days, but, yes, you can adapt to changes, or in this case, a new diet, if you consistently and consciously see to it that you embrace the changes in your life. I would like you to treat the first 21 days in the Paleo Diet as a honeymoon phase. Think of these days as the beginning of a longer journey ahead—a journey to a healthier you!

Week 1

Congratulations! You are on your first week on the Paleo Challenge. I'm pretty sure you're well-motivated right now to take on the diet and I would like you to use this as a leverage so you can go through seven whole days with ease.

Day 1: Do a Pantry Inventory

This is obviously the first thing you have to do should you decide to commit to the diet and jump in this Paleo challenge. As you can see in the previous chapter, I have listed down the types of foods you need to avoid in the diet and I'm quite sure that you have these lying around in your kitchen. Do you have cereals in your cupboard? What about hotdogs and sausages? Do you love drinking soda and all sorts of sugary drinks—well, I got news for you. All of them must go.

OK. I'll cut you some slack since it's only the first day in the challenge. You have the option to dump the foods not in the Paleo Diet one at a time. But believe me, as long as you're not letting go of these ugly carbs, sugar-laden pastries, and unhealthy processed food in your kitchen, the more you will be tempted to go back on munching on them. So if you do have the courage to do so, I would really recommend for you to clear your stock with any food that are not Paleo friendly. Refined sugar, grains, and legumes all must go.

Also take this opportunity to clean your food storage and to have an inventory with what food you have left. Doing this will allow you to know which foods you're going to buy on your next visit to the supermarket.

Day 2: Go shopping!

Now that you're done purging your pantry, you must have almost nothing left in your food stock. The only logical thing to do next is to go shopping!

Oops! Before you rush to the nearest supermarket, what you need to do is to know and list down which paleo foods you need to buy. *Why do you need to do this, you ask?* Having a list of what you need to buy lowers the risk of you buying "extra" items that are not included in the Paleo Diet. Plus, this will also save you from wasting money because you are only going to buy ingredients that you will need for your Paleo meals.

If there are any shopping tips that I have learned since I decided to jump on this diet, it's these four things:

1. Planning is a must! I will never, and I say, never, go to the grocery without a list on hand or without any idea what I will cook for the days to come.

2. Stay away from the inner aisle. I discovered that most ingredients that I need (those that are fresh and healthy) are stored along the perimeter aisles of the grocery stores. It's very dangerous to venture in the center aisles because these are where the "goodies are".

3. Buy produce that are in season. This keeps my food budget within the ideal range. Of course, when these produce are in season, it means that there is a surplus in the supply, which also means they are sold cheaper during this time.

4. Buy in bulk. If I can and if I have the budget to, I stock up on food like meat. Not many realize this, but buying in bulk saves you some money and also time.

Day 3: Eat at Least Two Paleo Meals Daily

This is another hall pass that I will allow you to have. If you're having hard time preparing and eating Paleo dishes for all your meals, then you can at least start to challenge yourself to eating two paleo meals daily for the rest of the week. This is the beauty of the Paleo Diet, you don't have to go cold turkey with your former diet so you can immediately adapt to Paleo meal plan. Remember that you're aiming to change not only how you eat, but your whole lifestyle. That's why if it's carefully introducing Paleo meals to your diet works for you, then by all means, do it. However, I would want you to remember that the end goal is to fully adapt to the Paleo lifestyle in order for you to reap its benefits.

Day 4: Eat Breakfast Starting from Today

Whether or not you believe that breakfast is the most important meal of the day or not, eating breakfast for any type of diet is beneficial to the body, period. Remember that our body needs fuel for it to function properly. Without filling up with fuel, we won't have the energy to face the hectic day ahead.

However, you need to take note that you must have quality fuel when filling up for the day. What I mean is that you should make it a point that your breakfast does not consist of sugary cereals, but by the perfect energy driving foods which are protein, good gats, and complex carbs. You can use the recipes in the following chapter to make your breakfast dishes with.

Day 5: Make Your Own Paleo Snacks

Do you always have the tendency to crave food in between meals? If you're on the Paleo Diet for a couple of days now, you might notice that your bouts with hunger are diminishing every day. That's because Paleo meals are rich in protein and fiber which makes you feel satiated for longer periods of time. However, if you're really hungry or is itching to munch on snacks in between meals, luckily, there are snacks that are Paleo-friendly.

Of course, I would recommend for you to make the snacks yourself to have control over what you eat. Just make sure that you're making the right choices when it comes to the food you will snack on. This means that cookies, muffins, and energy bars are out of the question. If you need recipes for snacks, I have listed down some for you in Chapter 7.

Day 6: Read about Meal Prepping

Are you now having a hard time making your own meals? Do you feel like you don't have enough time to eat breakfast and to at least eat two Paleo dishes a day? Then, my challenge for you today is to learn about meal prepping.

When you learn to prepare meals for the days ahead, you are able to save time, money, and also be able to stick to the Paleo meal plan. So I encourage you to take the time today to read references on how you can apply meal prepping in the Paleo Diet.

Some simple things you can do is to pre-cook protein sources, hard boil a batch of eggs that you will eat for a few days, or basically, prepare any foods that will require advance preparation. Of course, besides cooking in batches, you also need to know your portions depending on your dietary needs and health goals. This also means that you should invest in food-grade and freezer safe containers for you to store your prepared food with.

Day 7: Exercise!

If you decide to go on the Paleo Diet to lose weight, then I've got news for you. Those pounds aren't going to shed effectively without partnering the healthy diet with exercise. This is the same if your goal is to be athletic and agile like the cavemen were.

Good thing, just like the meals in the Paleo Diet, the physical activities that you are recommended to do aren't too complicated. It could be as simple as physically moving a little bit more than you used to.

Of course, it would be great if you incorporated in your daily routine at least 30 minutes of exercise such as brisk walking, jogging, or cycling. Doing this overtime will allow to reap the many benefits of regular exercise such as improving your immune system, keeping your heart healthy, improving your mobility and agility, as well as preventing diabetes, and stroke. Obviously, regular physical activity partnered with a healthy diet is always synonymous with losing weight. So, you're practically achieving a number of goals when you eat healthy and exercise.

Week 2

Wow! You made it this far! I am hoping that after a week on the Paleo Diet, you can already feel the changes in your body. You still might experience some road bumps here and there, but hey, you're getting there! It is the second week of the 21-Day Paleo Challenge, so I encourage you to press on and continue with the excellent work!

Day 8: Create a 7-Day Paleo Meal Plan

It's your eighth day on the diet so you're probably bored of the baby steps you made last week, that's why today, I am going to challenge you to make an entire week's worth of Paleo Meal Plan. You were already given enough excuses the previous week, it's time to man up and really take on the challenge.

Maybe you survived the whole week without drafting a meal plan, but believe me, making one will make things easier for you. It will also enable you to overcome the challenges of going back to your old diet.

To give you an idea of what a well-rounded Paleo meal looks like, all you need to remember are these three basic rules below:

- Aim for filling half of your plate with a huge pile of vegetables.
- Eat a one to two palm-sized protein every main meal, or 3-4 eggs.
- Include healthy fat in your meals

You can also use the recipes in the following chapters to plan your meals with.

Day 9: Get Your Measurements

Do you want to have the motivation to keep going with the Paleo Diet to lose weight despite the temptations lurking around? Know your measurements! Take the courage to face the truth and get the right numbers. Weigh in, measure your waist, and know what other numbers need to go down (for example, your blood pressure) and write everything down! Having a record of these things will help remind you how far you've accomplished since going into the diet and how much work you still need to do in order to achieve ideal or healthy numbers.

Day 10: Increase Your Physical Activity

By now, I hope that you've already incorporated in your routine a regular physical work out. As this is your second week in the diet, I would encourage you to take things up a notch and further increase your physical activity. Although you have a regular schedule for exercise, I would recommend you to increase your movement at home or at work. For example, parking your car further away from your office building to walk a few steps more every day or ditching the elevator and opting for the stairs instead. At home, you can do a "semi" spring cleaning or other errands that will require you to move more—all these little things contribute a lot!

Day 11: Find Your Support System

Hang in there! You're halfway in the 21 Day Paleo Challenge. You've come this far so don't ever think of cheating and backing down. If you want to keep on moving and fully adapt to the lifestyle, my challenge for you today is to find your support system by joining a Paleo community.

You can do this by simply going on line and looking for groups who are also into the diet like you. If you could, find support groups within your community. With these support systems, you are able to learn things from other people who are going through the same struggles and achieving the same goals like you.

Day 12: Say Goodbye to Dairy!

As you already know, the Paleo Diet limits the consumption of dairy food items. And if you haven't still fully given up on these types of food, then I challenge you to say *adios* to them (or at least some of them) today.

Although as infants, we got our nourishment and beneficial nutrients from our mother's milk, consuming dairy from another source (like animals) is believed by the proponents of the Paleo Diet as bad for our health.

First of all, humans are the only mammals who get milk from other animals. Since cow's milk isn't naturally designed for our body, some may experience intolerance or allergic reaction from drinking an animal's milk. Also, another problem with milk is that it has high level of carbs which means it is insulin promoting that can aggravate issues related to weight and controlling insulin.

If you decide to consume some dairy products, you may opt to choose products that are more Paleo-friendly. Some examples of dairy that you can include in your diet are organic or grass-fed, full fat yogurt, butter, kefir, cheese, and some clarified butter or ghee.

Day 13: Learn About Detox

Maybe you feel like under the weather right now and you're not seeing the changes in your body after a few days in the Paleo Diet. Maybe, you're even experiencing some headaches, fatigue, increased urination, or increased thirst. You don't have to worry when you're experiencing these things because these are symptoms of your body cleaning itself with all the toxins that it accumulated over the years.

Now that you're eating clean, whole foods, and there are no harmful chemicals that are disrupting your organs, and your body is now going through detoxification. A lot of Paleo Dieters undergo this detox phase starting on the third day of the diet up to the third week, so you don't have to worry if you're not feeling anything other than the symptoms of detoxification.

Of course, I would encourage you to learn more about this so you can keep check whether the discomfort you're feeling is nothing or something to worry about.

Day 14: Get Enough Sleep

Again it's not just your diet that you're trying to improve, it's your over-all lifestyle. Time and time again, getting enough quality sleep is very important if you want to stay in shape and be healthy. Unfortunately, most of us have forgotten the importance of sleep. That's why starting today, I challenge you to get a good night sleep as often as you could. Some of the benefits of getting enough sleep are mental clarity, boosts mood and energy, increase in productivity, improves athletic performance, strengthens the immune system, and reduces stress.

Week 3

You deserve a pat on the back! Great job for getting through two weeks of the Paleo Lifestyle! You're almost done with the 21-day challenge so just hang in there!

Day 15: Go out and say hello to Mr. Sun

The first challenge this week is quite easy—go outside and get some fresh air! If you've been spending time at the gym for your exercise routine, I say, change that routine this week and try running outside. Or even better, why not go on a hike?

A research from the University of Essex found that going outdoors and being one with nature makes exercise easier and it also makes you look forward to your next workout. Also, another study published in the Journal of Experimental Psychology found that spending time outdoors where there are trees, grass, and clean air increases one's concentration skills and creativity. Being under the sun also increases your intake of the Vitamin D that is essential for bone growth, cell growth, and prevention of inflammation.

Day 16: Ditch a Bad Habit

You've been doing great so far. You've turned away from eating unhealthy foods, started cooking healthy and also incorporated some physical activity in your daily routine; what else can you not overcome, right? So today, I challenge you to think of a habit that you think you can change. Is it smoking? Indulging in alcohol? Or spending too much time in front of the TV?

Again, you've come along this far, so I'm pretty sure you have it in you to overcome this habit.

Day 17: Push! Go All Out on Your Exercise

Never allow yourself to stagnate and keep challenging yourself for more. Yes, you've been doing cardio for over two weeks now, but how about introducing other routines in your workouts? If you're still experiencing the effects of detox in your body, I'd advise to delay this challenge when you're feeling better.

But if not, and if your head is really in the game, then I challenge you to push yourself further in your exercises. CrossFit is one of the most popular fitness programs in the Paleo Diet and you might want to consider doing it—of course, with the help of a trainer. This type of program helps promote overall fitness and will indeed release the inner caveman in you. But do remember that it takes months of training before you get to enjoy and see the benefits of CrossFit, yes, training is hard and very challenging, but it's very worth it.

Day 18: Go Crazy with Cooking

Put all the things you've learned about meal prepping into practice. If today is a weekend and you have free time, then perfect! Today you are going to go crazy in the kitchen. Make your Paleo Meal plan and plot it around what food you have available and how many batches of food you will make. Personally, when I have the time to cook, I see to it that I cook my meals in double portions because this allows me to store leftovers in the freezer so I have ready-to-go meals on hectic days.

Day 19: Get Your Loved Ones on Board

It's time to go through the Paleo journey with your family or friends. Of course, it will be more fun and easier for you to adopt to this lifestyle if the whole of your household is in the diet too.

If you're the one in charge of what is place on the dinner table, then good for you, because you have the power to "switch" your old meals to Paleo-friendly meals. If you have kids, you can slowly substitute their favorite sugary sweets to delicious Paleo treats.

Again, planning ahead is the key to this so make sure you prepare ahead. Look for recipes that you know the members of your family will love. Just keep on introducing the Paleo Diet to them and they'll eventually adapt to it easily.

Day 20: Say Goodbye to Ugly Carbs

Like what I mentioned in the previous chapters, carbs are ugly because they are making you unhealthy. Now as you move closer to the end of the 21-Day Paleo Challenge, I would like you to make a vow of turning your back on ugly carbs forever—because again, they substantially couldn't be good for our health.

Don't get me wrong, our body still needs carbohydrates, but you have to choose the good ones to be included in your diet. *How do you know if it's good carbs?* Here are some indications of how:

- If they are high in fiber (these are generally considered the healthy type of carbs)

- These are mostly vegetables and fruits (like berries)

- These are foods with low glycemic index which means they only increase blood sugar and insulin gradually, which is good.

- And again, you can check Chapter 2 to see which type of carb sources are best for your meals.

Day 21: Reward Yourself

Today is a good day because you finished three whole weeks of the Paleo Lifestyle. This day, all you have to do is to reward yourself for getting this far. But take note, what I mean by reward is not indulging on the foods that you avoided these past few days—Hey, you've gotten this far, do you really want to go back to square one?

What I mean is that you should go treat yourself with something that will make you feel good. For example, a day at the spa, or simply buying the shoes you've been eyeing for weeks. Celebrate because you're well on your way to a healthier you!

The 21-Day Paleo Challenge is over, but the road is still long. I just hope that these challenges have helped you adapt to the lifestyle easier. If you must, I encourage you to create a challenge of your own so that you will have goals to work on and look forward to.

Chapter 5

Paleo-Approved Breakfast Recipes

Recipe #1: Crab Omelet

Ingredients:

3 eggs

1 tsp. water

2 tsp. canola oil

1 small onion (diced)

1 small tomato (diced)

1 tsp. fresh basil

Salt and fresh black pepper

¼ lb. crab meat (shredded especially the claw part)

Remember processed food is not a Paleo-friendly food. So buy fresh crab.

Procedure:

1. To cook the crab, boil 1 liter of water in the pot. When the water starts to boil, put in the whole crab and cook

for about 15 to 20 minutes. Remove the crab from the pan and rinse under running water to stop the cooking process and let it cool. Start cracking it and remove the meat out from the shell and shred.

2. In a medium non-stick pan heat 1 tsp. canola oil over a medium heat.

3. Add in crab, onion and tomato and fresh basil and add a dash of salt of pepper to taste. Set it aside.

4. In a bowl, place the eggs and add 1 tsp. of water (this will make the texture of the egg fluffy). Beat the mixture using a fork or an egg beater until well blended.

5. In the pan add the remaining canola oil and put in the beaten egg mixture, when the base of the omelet starts to firm up, but still has small amount of raw egg on top, add in the crab – tomato- onion mixture.

6. Carefully ease the edges of the omelet using a spatula, then fold in half.

7. Place in a platter and serve.

Recipe #2: Yummy Paleo Pancake

Ingredients:

3 eggs, beaten

4 mashed bananas (any variety)

1 small sized apple (peeled and diced)

1 ½ tsp. cinnamon powder

2 ½ tbsp. almond butter

Walnuts (optional)

½ tsp. pure vanilla extract

1 tbsp. (or more) grass-fed butter

Procedure:

1. Beat 3 eggs in a bowl and add in mashed bananas.
2. Add in diced apple, walnuts and blend in the banana and egg mixture evenly.
3. Add the cinnamon powder, almond butter, and vanilla extract. Mix in the pancake batter.
4. Over medium heat, pre-heat a non-stick pan add melt butter, and then pour small amount of the pancake batter into the pan.
5. Cook until small bubbles appear on top, but golden brown and firm at the bottom, (for about 3 to 4 minutes). Flip and cook the other side.
6. Top with fresh fruits instead of pan cake syrup to that perfect guilt- free pancake!

Enjoy a healthy breakfast!

Recipe #3: Veggies and Egg Cups

Ingredients:

6 organic eggs

1 medium sized white onion

1 cup broccoli florets (chopped)

1 cup zucchini (chopped)

1 cup fresh asparagus (chopped)

1 cup spinach (chopped)

A dash of kosher salt and freshly cracked black pepper to taste

Procedure:

1. Preheat the oven to 300F. Beat eggs in a mixing bowl and in a dash of salt and pepper; then stir in the chopped veggies.

2. Prepare porcelain ramekins by brushing it with oil. (*If you do not have a ramekin dish, you can use muffin pans*)

3. Transfer the egg mixture into the ramekin dish and bake for 20-35 minutes or until the eggs are set.

4. Remove from heat and let sit for 10 minutes before serving. Top it celery.

Recipe #4: Paleo Hamburger *Gustoso!*

Ingredients

6 eggs

3 strips of cooked bacon strips

½ lb. ground grass-fed beef

1/8 tsp. of nutmeg

1/8 tsp. of pepper

A dash of sea salt to taste

1 tsp. of fennel seeds

1 tbsp. of olive oil

Procedure:

1. In a bowl, mix together ground beef, fennel seeds, nutmeg, salt and pepper.
2. Shape it into patties and set aside.
3. Place a skillet on low to medium heat.
4. In the heated skillet scramble the eggs shaping it into several uneven circles, flip on other side to cook. Set aside.
5. In the same pan fry beef patties until golden brown or for 4 to 5 minutes.

6. Get cooked patties from the pan.

7. Use the scrambled egg as your bread layering it with patties and bacon in between.

Enjoy your carb free, hamburger gustoso!

Recipe #5: Homemade Paleo Corned Beef

Ingredients

4 cups corned beef (cooked and chopped)

2 cups radishes (cut into quarters)

1 medium sized onion (chopped)

2 garlic cloves (minced)

¾ cup beef broth

Salt and pepper to add flavor

1 tbsp. olive oil

Procedure:

1. Over medium to high fire, heat the skillet drizzled with 1 tbsp. olive oil.

2. Put in onions and sauté for 5 minutes, add in the radishes and cook for another 5 minutes.

3. Add in the garlic and continue sautéing for another minute.

4. Pour in the beef broth and then loosely cover the pan. Simmer until the radishes are tender and cooked.

5. Add in the corned beef and mix well.

6. Dash with salt and pepper to taste.

Recipe #6: Paleo Breakfast Bake

Ingredients

3 tbsp. bacon fat

1 lb. steak, cut into bite sized pieces

1 green bell pepper, small-sized chopped

1 small red bell pepper, chopped

1 large-sized sweet potatoes, cut 1" cubes

1 small tomato, sliced

4 eggs (beaten)

Kosher salt and black pepper to taste

Procedure:

1. Set oven to 370F

2. Heat up the bacon fat in a pan over medium to high heat.

3. Add in steak and cook until it turns brown. Set aside.

4. In the same pan sauté the green and red bell peppers and onions for 2 to 3 minutes.

5. Put in sweet potatoes and sautéing in all together until tender for 8 to 10 minutes.

6. Put the steak in a baking pan and stir everything together.

7. Using the back of a spoon make a small indention to the mixtures.

8. Pour the beaten eggs into the indentations.

9. Add in tomatoes on top of the eggs.

10. Add salt and pepper to give a flavorful taste.

11. Put the skillet in the oven and bake for 10 minutes, or until done.

Recipe #7: Healthy Cucumber Sandwich

Ingredients

4 slices of turkey breast (you may also use chicken as substitute for turkey)

5 slices of crunchy bacon

1 medium sized cucumber

Dijon mustard

Spreadable garlic and herbs

Procedure:

1. Cut the cucumber into half and scooping out all the seeds.

2. Evenly spread the garlic and herb on the cucumber

3. Meanwhile, cook the turkey slices in a pan with ¼ cup of water. Season with a dash of kosher salt.

4. Remove from the heat when the turkey slices are done and let it cool down for a bit.

5. Arrange the turkey slices on top of the hollow cucumber add mustard and crunchy bacon bites.

6. Place the other half on top to make a sandwich.

A sandwich without bread that is an appetizing Paleo food!

Chapter 6

The Caveman's Meal Recipes

Recipe #1: Tuna and Cabbage Medley

Ingredients for tuna:

6-8 pieces tuna fillets

3 tbsp. olive oil

1 large beaten egg

1 tsp. freshly ground pepper

½ cup cassava flour

¼ tsp. mustard powder

Sea salt to give flavor

Ingredients for sautéed cabbage:

1 head cabbage, sliced

1 tbsp. olive oil

½ cup chicken broth

1 cups cauliflower florets

5 cloves of garlic (chopped)

Procedure:

Tuna Preparation:

1. Mix cassava flour, freshly ground pepper, salt and powdered mustard in a small bowl and transfer it to an empty plate.

2. Dip tuna fillets one at a time in egg and dredge with flour mixture.

3. Fry for about 2 to 3 minutes on each or until golden brown.

4. Set aside.

Cabbage Preparation:

1. Place a large pan over a low to medium fire. Add in oil and heat.

2. Throw in the in chopped garlic and sauté for 2 minutes.

3. Add cauliflower florets and sauté for another 3 minutes.

4. Add in cabbage and continue sautéing. Do not over cook

5. Pour over chicken stock, simmering it for 1 more minute.

Serve the sautéed cabbage as your side dish for healthy tuna meal.

Recipe #2: Tenderloin Steak and Squash-Spinach Soup Combo

Ingredients:

Ingredients for steak:

1/2 lb. Tenderloin steak

½ tsp. kosher salt

½ tsp. ground pepper

A pinch of dried thyme

1 tbsp. olive oil

Squash Spinach soup

1 lb. squash

½ lb. of fresh spinach

Kosher salt and pepper to taste

Small onion (roughly chopped)

3 cloves of garlic (chopped)

4 cups of water

Procedure:

1. Prepare your soup first. In a heated medium sized skillet, sauté garlic, and onion.

2. Add in squash and sauté for 3 more minutes.

3. Add 3 cups of water and cook the squash until very tender.

4. Add in spinach and cook for another 3 minutes.

5. Turn off heat and let it cool for about 5 minutes.

6. After 5 minutes, transfer the mixture into a food processor or a blender.

7. Blend well until you produce a puree.

8. Bring back to pan and the remaining cup of water (or adding more depending on the consistency you prefer) and let it simmer for 1 minute.

9. Prepare the tenderloin beef. Season it with salt, pepper and thyme. Set aside.

10. Heat olive oil in a cast iron skillet over a medium heat. Put in the meat and cook uncovered for 6 to 15 minutes on each side or depending on your desired doneness. (Medium rare 6 to10 minutes. Well done 12 to 15 minutes.)

11. Throw in your veggies as side dish; like sautéed carrots, zucchini, cucumber, turnip, green and red bell

peppers and many more.

Serve tenderloin steak together with the squash spinach soup to have a complete meal.

Recipe #3: Spicy Chicken Guacamole and Mango Salad

Ingredients

2 to 4 cups of shredded chicken breast

2 medium sized mango, peeled and diced

2 medium sized guacamole, diced

1 head of romaine lettuce (chopped)

1 tsp. of chili powder

½ tsp. of cumin

Salt and pepper to taste

Procedure:

1. Place the romaine lettuce into a large bowl.
2. In a separate bowl, put the shredded chicken and add a 5 tbsp. of water.
3. Cook for 15 to 20 seconds in a microwave oven over a

medium-high heat.

4. After cooking, mix in the cumin and chili powder.

5. Put the chicken with cumin and chili powder into the large bowl of lettuce.

6. Top it with guacamole and mango.

7. Enjoy your meal. No need to add a dressing it is appetizing as it is.

Recipe #4: Calvolfiore Riso

Craving for "rice"? Here is a substitute!

Ingredients:

2 heads of cauliflower

1/8 tsp. ground black pepper

4 cloves garlic (chopped)

4 tbsp. bacon fat

½ cup chopped fresh cilantro

1 medium sized white onion, chopped (about 1 cup)

½ tsp. kosher salt

Make sure to follow the instructions step by step for a satisfying "rice" recipe.

Procedure:

1. Chop the cauliflowers. Toss into the food processor or a blender until the cauliflower pieces are the shape and size of rice. Be careful not to over blend.

2. Do them by batches. When you're done set aside the chopped cauliflower.

3. Heat a medium-sized skillet over low to medium fire. Sauté the garlic and onion in oil for 1 minute. Add in the chopped cauliflower mixing it well.

4. Then add the salt and pepper to flavor, sauté it for 5 more minutes or until the cauliflower is slightly tender.

5. Serve in a bowl and add some freshly chopped cilantro!

You may add in your favorite Paleo veggies like chopped and blanched carrots, bell pepper, zucchini, cucumber, beets and a lot more. You may also add paprika or cumin for that tangy taste.

Recipe #5: Paleo Pasta

Use a peeler or spiral vegetable slicer for making your "pasta"

Ingredients

6 medium zucchini

5 tbsp. pesto

½ lb. fresh grape tomatoes (cut into halves)

Sea salt and freshly ground black pepper, to add flavor

Light olive oil

Dried thyme or basil

Almond nuts (chopped)

Procedure:

1. With the use of a peeler or the spiral vegetable cutter, slice the zucchini lengthwise just like a noodle, stop when you reach the seeds.

2. Turn it on the anther side and continue the process. If you are using vegetable peeler, slice it some more into thin diagonal strips to make look more look like spaghetti.

3. Heat a medium-sized pan over a low to medium fire. Add olive oil toss in the "pasta". Cook it for 5 to 7 minutes stirring it continuously.

4. Add a dash salt and ground pepper for flavor.

5. Remove from heat, mix the pesto, tossing until well coated.

6. Top with tomatoes, almond nuts, dried thyme or basil.

Now you have a carb and gluten free pasta! Bon a petit!

Recipe #6: Fruity Pork Chops

Ingredients:

5 bone in pork chops

4 whole apples (medium sliced)

½ cup pork bone broth (you may also use chicken of beef broth)

fresh parsley (chopped)

6 cloves of garlic (minced)

coarse black pepper and sea salt to taste

½ tsp. garlic powder

½ tsp. onion powder for flavor

3 tbsp. ghee

Procedure:

1. Heat a large sized frying pan over medium fire. Throw in the garlic, parsley and broth and let it simmer for 2 minutes.

2. Flavor the pork chops with onion powder, garlic powder, salt and black pepper.

3. Place the chops in a skillet and cook for 4 to 6 minutes or until brown spooning some of the garlic broth over the meat. Flip over and continue to cook until done.

4. In a separate frying pan, melt the ghee and sauté apples over a low to medium heat until it is tender.

5. Transfer the cooked apples into the other pan with pork chops and marinate together for 5 minutes to blend in the flavors.

6. Serve on a platter spooning over the pork chop broth with the apples on top.

Recipe #7 Salmon in Coconut Cream Sauce

Ingredients:

1 ½ pounds salmon fillet

¾ cup full fat coconut milk

3 tbsp. coconut toil

¼ freshly ground pepper

1 large diced shallot

4 gloves minced garlic

¼ tsp. kosher salt

1 medium lemon zest

½ cup lemon juice

3 tbsp. freshly chopped basil

Procedure:

1. Preheat oven to 350F.

2. Place salmon fillet in a baking dish, sprinkle it with salt and freshly ground pepper on both sides.

3. Heat a pan over medium fire. Add the coconut oil, garlic and shallots. Cook for few more minutes until the shallots have softened.

4. Add in coconut milk, lemon juice and lemon zest and bring to a low boil.

5. Add in basil and reduce the heat.

6. Pour the coconut milk mixture over the salmon, baking it uncovered for about 10 to 20 minutes or until done.

Enjoy your healthy salmon meal!

Chapter 7

Irresistible Paleo-Friendly Snacks

Recipe #1: The Caveman's Pizza

Ingredients

1 ½ cups of almond flour

4 tbsp. almond butter

3 large – sized egg (beaten)

½ tsp. kosher salt

4 tsp. olive oil

1 large- sized white onion (diced)

5 medium-sized mushroom, (sliced)

1 sausage cut into thick slices

10 strips of bacon cooked and crushed

1 large green bell pepper (diced)

1 cup tomato sauce, marinara sauce with no salt added

½ tsp. oregano

1 cup cherry tomatoes sliced in half

Procedure:

1. Preheat the oven to 350F.

2. In a small bowl mix almond flour, egg, butter, salt and combine well.

3. Brush a baking sheet with half of the olive oil, and pour the mixture over it, and make a ¼ thin crust and cook in the oven for 10 minutes.

4. While waiting for the crust, heat a large skillet over a medium fire. Add olive oil, white onions, sausages, and mushrooms and cook until brown. Remove from pan and set aside.

5. In the same pan, throw in the garlic and green pepper and sauté for a few minutes or until tender. Do not overcook.

6. Take out the crust from the oven and generously spread the marinara sauce on it. Top with sausage and sautéed veggies.

7. Sprinkle with oregano, and place in the oven for 25 to 30 minutes.

8. Remove from the oven when cooked.

9. Top with sliced tomatoes and crushed bacon.

10. Serve.

Recipe #2: Raspberry and Almond Muffin Cups

Ingredients:

2 cups almond flour

1 tsp. baking powder

1 tsp. baking soda

1 tsp. almond extract

4 large eggs (beaten)

2 cups almond butter

½ cup raw honey

½ cup silvered almonds

½ coconut oil

2 cups raspberries

½ tsp. salt

Procedure:

1. Preheat your oven to 350 F.
2. In a large bowl combine all of the dry ingredients together. Set aside.

3. In another bowl combine almond butter, egg, almonds, honey, almond extract, and coconut oil.

4. Gradually mix in with the dry ingredients.

5. Mix the fresh raspberries.

6. Slightly grease muffin pan with coconut oil, or line it with paper muffin liners then scoop batter evenly into 8-10 muffins cups.

7. Bake for 15-20 minutes. Watch muffins to be sure they do not overcook.

Recipe #3: A Perfect Fresh Fruit Salad

Ingredients:

1 medium sized oranges (peeled and diced)

1 medium sized apple (diced)

1 medium sized peach (chopped)

1 lb. black grapes (cut into halves)

1 lb. green grapes (cut into halves)

½ cup walnut and almonds (chopped)

½ tsp. cinnamon powder

Procedure:

1. Combine all fruits in a bowl.
2. Sprinkle with chopped nuts and cinnamon.

Recipe #4: The Paleo Banana Carrot Muffin

Ingredients:

4 cups almond flour

4 tsp. baking soda

1 salt

2 tsp. cinnamon powder

2 cups pitted dates

6 medium sized bananas

6 large eggs

2 tsp. apple cider vinegar

½ cup coconut oil

2 large carrots (grated)

1 cup walnut (finely chopped)

Procedure:

1. Pre heat oven to 350F

2. In a large bowl, mix baking soda, salt and cinnamon.

3. Blend the pitted dates, bananas, eggs, oil and vinegar in a food processor.

4. In a large bowl transfer the mixture from the food processor to the dry ingredients mixing it thoroughly.

5. Fold in grated carrots and nuts.

6. Scoop mixture into the paper lined muffin tins.

7. Bake 25 minutes, or until done. To test, insert a toothpick at the center of the muffin, when the toothpick comes out clean, then your muffin is done!

Recipe #5: Crunchy Zucchini

Ingredients:

3 cups zucchini

3 large eggs

Salt and pepper to taste

2 tbsp. bacon grease

2 tbsp. coconut flour (sifted)

Procedure:

1. Using a peeler shred the zucchini thinly, stopping when you reach the seeds. Turn zucchini to the other side and do the same procedure. Dry with paper towel to remove excess water). Set aside.

2. Beat eggs in a large bowl.

3. Add coconut flour into the beaten eggs, and mix together.

4. Flavor the shredded zucchini with salt and pepper and combine it with the egg mixture.

5. Place a large pan over a medium- low heat. When the pan is already hot, add bacon grease to coat the pan.

6. Spoon in the mixture into the pan. Depending on the size of fritters you like.

7. Fry until golden brown and crispy.

8. Serve warm.

Recipe #6: Dates Wrapped in Crispy Bacon

Ingredients

10 slices of bacon cut into half

20 pitted dates

20 almonds

20 pieces toothpick

Procedure:

1. Preheat oven to 350 F
2. With the use of a knife open up the dates
3. Stuff one almond inside each date.
4. Wrap each date with a bacon slice. Securing it with a toothpick.
5. On a shallow baking pan, put the bacons with dates and bake for 6 minutes.
6. Turnover and bake for another 6 minutes or until bacon is crispy.
7. Serve it warm or cold.

Recipe #7: Chocolate Banana Muffin

Ingredients:

1 cup mashed banana

3 large eggs

½ tsp. vanilla extract

3 tbsp. raw honey

¼ cup coconut oil

¼ cup coconut flour

½ baking soda

½ tsp. salt

¼ cup unsweetened cocoa powder

¼ cup semi-sweet chocolate chips

Procedure:

1. Preheat the oven to 350 F.

2. Place paper baking cups into a muffin pan.

3. Combine the mashed banana, beaten egg, vanilla extract, and coconut oil, in a mixing bowl and mix all the ingredients well.

4. Add in coconut oil, baking soda, salt and cocoa powder. Mix and fold well until all ingredients are evenly blended.

5. Spoon in the batter into each paper cup.

6. Sprinkle the chocolate chips on top.

7. Bake for 15 to 20 minutes or until done. To test if it is done, insert a toothpick in the middle of the muffin if it comes out mostly clean, then it is done!

8. Let it cool and enjoy your chocolatey muffin!

Conclusion

Paleo Diet or the Caveman's Diet has been proven to be effective by many individuals who had struggles with physical appearance because of their excess weight. However, Paleo Diet is not only for people who have weight issues, but also to those who want to be healthy.

Following the Paleo Lifestyle at first, might be tough and frustrating mainly because you have been used to be chomping "junk food" for many years. But committing to this diet and putting your heart out into trying it will surely give you positive results.

I'd also like to remind you that aside from these healthy foods that you will consume, exercise should also be included in your daily routine. Sufficient sleep and managing stress as much as possible is a sure way in achieving your goals like a desired "bikini bod" and optimum health.

Do not waste time any further! Give the 21-day Paleo Challenge a shot and you'll surely reap its benefits in no time!

Check Out Other Books

Go here to check out other related books that might interest you:

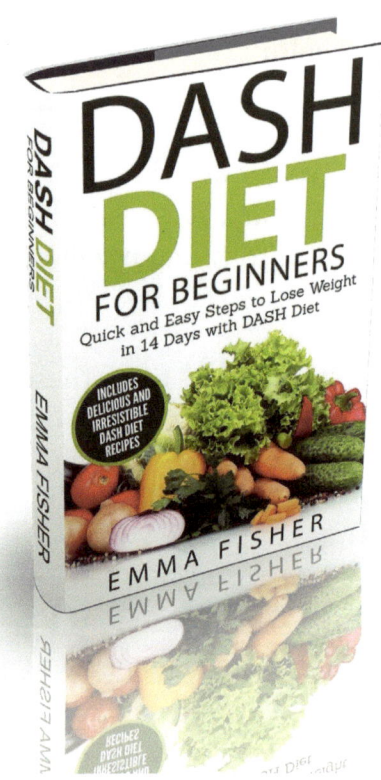

The DASH Diet for Beginners

Quick and Easy Steps to Lose Weight in 14 Days with DASH Diet

http://www.amazon.com/dp/B0127KQQ0I

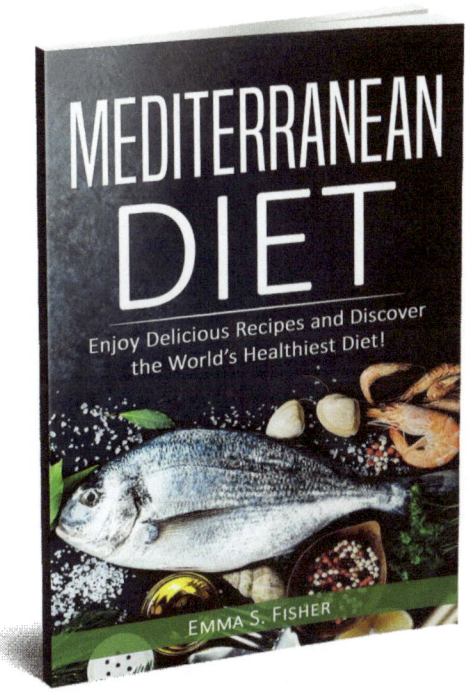

Mediterranean Diet: Enjoy 20 Delicious Recipes and Discover the World's Healthiest Diet!

https://www.amazon.com/dp/B01LXC2RLO

www.ingramcontent.com/pod-product-compliance
Lightning Source LLC
Chambersburg PA
CBHW040323010626
45792CB00024B/2103